+ BONUS: 50 Days Action Plan

ESCAPE THE BINGE CYCLE

BED: Proven Methods to Stop Binge Eating and Lose Weight

Kobenan Georges

INTRODUCTION

Dear reader,

Welcome to the world of binge eating, finding yourself, and getting better.

People have been struggling silently with eating disorders for a long time, and binge eating is among the most common.

As you read this book, you'll learn new things about binge eating, its causes, and recovery strategies.

Recovery may be a lengthy and arduous, but it is also full of hope and promise.

With my book, you'll learn useful tips and strategies to help you figure out why you binge eat and how to stop.

We'll also help you come up with a good plan to stop. You will also learn about the power of mind over binge, self-identity, and the science behind overcoming this disorder.

This book isn't just a collection of facts; it's also a life-changing guide that will help you get back in charge of your life and stop binge eating.

I'm glad to be a part of your journey, and I'm sure that the information, advice, and motivation in this book will help you become a healthier, happier person.

Thank you for choosing my book. I hope it will help you find yourself and heal on your way to self-discovery.

WHEN OUR SOULS ARE EMPTY

When our souls are empty, we want to fill our bodies.

We've all been there. You could put the plate down when you're full enough and still be fine.

You know that if you take another bite, you'll feel a little too full, but you do it anyway. That first bite leads to more.

You used to try to eat until you were full, but now you try to eat everything on your plate...and even more.

You're eating more quickly than you used to as if the food will go away if you don't eat it right away.

You want more flavour but can't tell what's in the food. You don't even think about food much anymore. You Eat it until it's gone from your plate, and you'll still want more.

It's not about the food or hunger anymore. Its now about filling your body up.

It's about how the different tastes and textures make your mouth feel.

It's about filling a craving for food and eating until you feel numb.

You don't even know why you're eating and already know you'll regret it. You feel sick, and part of you wants to stop, but the other half doesn't care.

It's never really about the food when you binge. It's about how you feel.

- Boredom
- Loneliness
- Frustration
- Anger
- Stres

The reasons we give ourselves to binge are really crazy. Like, really, where did all this creativity come from?

You tell yourself, "I'll start your healthy diet tomorrow." You say this as convincingly as a thief caught in the act.

You don't care, so you believe the white lie you tell yourself about your second piece of white cake, which you bought for tomorrow's guests but said you wouldn't eat. Oops.

You tell yourself, "You know what? I work so hard. I deserve this."

You come up with every reason why this eating binge is fine.

This has been a hard week.

Today, you ate well.

The last time you went out to dinner, you didn't have dessert.

All these are excuses you tell yourself as you dig deeper into your cabinets, looking for something to eat to satisfy your never-ending hunger.

We put food in our stomachs, where the solar plexus chakra is. This shows that there is an imbalance.

The solar plexus chakra controls how we feel about ourselves and how powerful we feel.

When we feel like we have no control over our lives, we focus on what we eat because it's the one thing we can always change.

Some people deal with this imbalance by not eating enough, while others do it too much. These responses come from the same feeling: you aren't whole yet.

When you don't eat enough, you show that your mind is stronger than your body. By not giving your body its most basic need, food, you feel strong because you have "beaten the system" by overcoming hunger, which is our most natural instinct.

When you eat too much, you're trying to fill yourself with love, fulfillment, community, or a sense of purpose. Something is missing inside you that you're trying to fill with food.

Most of the time, we learned to binge when we were young. Maybe a parent said you couldn't eat junk food, so you had to sneak away to get it. You got back to your parents by eating the "wrong" food. You may have felt like you were "beating the system" when you gorged on cupcakes when no one was looking. You ask yourself, "Did the tree really fall if no one heard it?"

But what started out as a "screw you" to your parents became a regular thing. You finally realize that binge eating hurts you, but it's too late to stop now.

That's because eating is now more than just eating; it's an experience. It's a way to protest. It might be one of the few times you get to be alone.

As a child, maybe the only time you had to yourself was late at night when you could get lost in a box of cookies in the kitchen. Even though you knew you shouldn't, it felt great to do it anyway.

Most of us didn't meditate when we were kids but were completely present when we ate. It was the only time of day when we felt like we were in our bodies, a feeling we craved. Eating makes us feel alive. It activates our senses.

When we eat too much, it's like we're looking for that feeling of being alive that food gives us. It's a primitive urge that fuels us to feed and feed and feed. In fact, it's a natural thing.

Our bodies were made to store as much fat as possible to keep us alive. It's a way to stay alive. That's why eating a lot of carbs and fats makes you feel so good. It's a reward from your brain for storing extra calories.

We don't live in the Ice Age, though. You don't need enough fat to make it through the winter. Even though your parents aren't telling you not to eat Halloween candy, you're still doing it.

You're an adult now. Your body is a choice you make. And there is no one else who can reap the rewards of it other than yourself. You aren't getting away with anything just because no one saw it. You are only hurting yourself.

Socializing

Some of us only binge when we are in the company of others. At birthday parties, weddings, and company events, there are always sweet and salty snacks and other foods we would never eat at home. So we overeat as much as we can.

Many think calories don't really count if we don't pay for the food. The food doesn't have to be in your kitchen to count.

There are many reasons why we binge when we're with other people.

1) We're happy.

2) We aren't being mindful.

3) We're less hard on ourselves.

4) It helps us get to know the people around us better.

Food is actually meant to be consumed socially. In all parts of the world, food is the center of social gatherings. Every night, families gather for dinner.

No one eats by himself. It's considered rude to eat without waiting for the rest of your tribe. Today, however, we often eat at our desks, on the go, or in front of our laptops.

So when we do see friends, it's for a meal. And we go HAM.

Think about it: when you want to hang out with someone, you probably ask if they want to meet for lunch, dinner, or even coffee and pastries. People don't say, "Let's get together under this beautiful tree and enjoy each other's company" as often as they used to. Though very lovely.

We have unconsciously linked getting together with people and eating. We relate the positive memories of birthdays, dinners, movie nights, and sleepovers with the food we ate during them.

Because we want to connect with other people so much, we often mistake that need for a pang of hunger for something we can satisfy more quickly, like food.

Our bodies and minds are linked. When we are stressed out or feeling alone, our minds want to go back to that happy place, and our bodies remember that they were eating food there, so they send us signals that they are hungry. What we really wanted was so much more than that.

Work and Binge

Food isn't just something we think about when we're with other people; it's also something we think about when we're alone. We often get hungry for snacks when we're working.

When working hard on something, the kitchen calls me every 10 minutes to satisfy another craving. I ignore it by making tea.

It's not because we are hungrier when working- it's because we subconsciously relate food as a break. We usually only take breaks to eat or use the bathroom.

When our minds need a break from the stress we've put them in, our bodies think, "I know what will get her away from that desk: food." Cue hunger signals."

Watch to see if you crave when you have a hard task. If so, your body is trying to tell you, "I don't want to be here right now." Instead of denying your body what it needs, listen to it by giving it a break and not using sugar to "relieve" your stress, which will make you feel worse.

Your body doesn't need a cookie; it must rest and heal. Go outside for a walk.

You'd be surprised at how regularly this occurs.

For example, binge eating disorder (BED) is the most common eating disorder there is. It affects about 3% of U.S. adults right now. Trusted Source

About 6% of the population has compulsive buying disorder, a more common Known Source.

It's also common for people, especially college students, to drink four or five drinks in less than two hours. Known Source

It turns out that drinking, eating, and shopping binges are all caused by the same things. All types of bingeing are unhealthy and irrational ways to deal with bad feelings.

When occasional overindulgence becomes a real problem, it causes feelings of helplessness, secrecy, shame, health problems, and social isolation.

When someone needs to binge alone or plans binges around work and social obligations, it's time to find out why.
Science and mental health

People often use "binge" to describe a meal bigger than planned or a long night of watching Netflix. But true binge eating is not the same as going back for seconds on mashed potatoes at

Thanksgiving or eating a lot of chips and dip at a Super Bowl party.

Genuine binge eating is recurrent and debilitating physically and emotionally.

It can cause high blood pressure, type 2 diabetes, high cholesterol, gallbladder disease, digestive problems, heart disease, and metabolic syndrome. It is often accompanied by anxiety and depression, which are hard to notice, just like binge eating.

Research shows that more than 20% of college-aged women have binged eaten and that a similar percentage of the general population will have a binge-eating disorder (BED) at some point in their lives.

1 Currently, about 60% of cases are found in women, and BED researchers think that less than 50% of all cases get the right treatment.

It is known that our brain's reward processes control appetite. In fact, scientists have found a neuron in our brains called PKC-delta that tells us when to stop eating. This neuron is in the amygdala.

This discovery has been taken to the next level by a new study that tried to find out if other neurons also affected our hunger.

The process used in the study is very complicated, but the results aren't hard to understand: when the mice eat, a neuron called HTR2a gets turned on, which makes them feel good and keep eating even when they're full.

Even more fascinating was the researcher's discovery of how the HTR2a neuron interacts with the PKC-delta neuron mentioned previously. Basically, they can both slow each other down.

Eating something terrible activates PKC-delta and tells us to stop eating, inhibiting HTR2-a cells. In the same way, eating something tasty turns on HTR2a cells, which tell us to keep eating and stop PKC-delta cells from working.

While the impact of these neurons is only shown in mice, researchers feel strongly that the same processes likely occur in humans.

If that's the case, it would greatly affect how people eat, and the reward system works.

For example, it could provide a neurological explanation for the moment discussed at the beginning of this article.

You may continue to eat something you enjoy even after you are full because HTR2a is activated, leading to feelings of reward that compel you to keep eating beyond satiation.

In layman's language, Brain imaging studies have identified two brain regions that appear to play a role in binge eating: the insula and the striatum.

The insula is a small, buried structure located in the cerebral cortex. It has been shown to play a key role in controlling how much food we eat, how much we weigh, and how hungry or full we feel.

Researchers have found that people with binge eating disorder have more activity in the insula when they see or smell food. This may be one reason they want to eat a lot quickly.

Part of the brain, called striatum, is responsible for motivation, processing rewards, and control their impulses.

Researchers have found that people with binge eating disorder may have changes in their striatum, making it hard to control how much food they eat. In particular, the striatum has been found to play a role in reinforcing binge-like eating behaviors; this may contribute to the difficulty of overcoming binge eating.

Yet, another region of the brain regulates appetite and body weight: the prefrontal cortex. It has been shown to help stop people from eating when they see food and stop them from eating when they don't feel like it.

Researchers have found that people with binge eating disorder may have less activity in their prefrontal cortex, making it hard to stop eating.

The available evidence suggests that alterations in these brain regions involved in reward processing, impulse control, and hunger regulation through mindfulness may play a role in developing and maintaining binge eating disorder.

Many experts have also found a link between bingeing and being absent, especially regarding emotions. People who are prone to compulsive behavior tend, in general, to have more difficulty understanding their feelings and handling stress.

There are many ways to help remedy the issue, such as mindfulness meditation and writing down emotions throughout the day.

When a binge feels imminent, Employ the THINK Method: ask whether these feelings are True, Helpful, Inspiring, Necessary, or Kind. For example, an impulse like, "I must buy that now," doesn't exactly fit the THINK bill.

Being aware of how you feel can help reduce stress, anxiety, and the bingeing that comes with it. You need to improve your mindfulness, which we will discuss in the next chapters.

As a binge eater, I learned that my brain constantly sought pleasure and reward. The reward center of my brain released the feel-good neurotransmitter dopamine when I saw or thought about tasty foods that were high in calories.

This reinforced the desire to consume more of those foods, leading to a vicious cycle of overeating.

Also, the pleasure centers had too much power over my prefrontal cortex, which is responsible for making decisions and keeping me in check. I couldn't stop wanting to eat, even though I knew it wasn't good for me.

During a binge, I felt like I had lost control as if I wasn't in charge of what I was doing.

This was because the part of my brain responsible for impulse control and inhibitory function, the orbitofrontal cortex, was being overridden by the pleasure centers.

Also, as I ate more and more, my levels of hormones like insulin and leptin, which control hunger and fullness, got out of whack.

This worsened my cravings and started a cycle of binging and feeling bad about myself afterward.

Overall, a binge eater's brain is a complicated mix of wanting pleasure, being impulsive, and having hormones that aren't working right. This leads to a repeated pattern of overeating.

MIND OVER BINGE

Studies shows that individuals who won't stop binging have abnormal brain dopamine levels.

Your brain is like a closest friend who would do whatever to ensure your safety.

This is sometimes done with a trick. Your brain is very good at tricking, diverting, digressing, sidestepping, shifting your focus, and even making things up to help you stay alive on this crazy, complicated place we call earth.

In the background, your brain is also working, so you can enjoy chocolate, sunshine, music, and whatever else makes you happy. Ultimately, it is made for your pleasure, making us more likely to binge.

And while it helps to know that your brain is on your side in the long run, it also helps to know when it uses questionable means to get to a good place. In a nutshell, your mind tricks you.

Living in your skull is the most sophisticated computational device known to man.

It is a very strong system that controls everything from what you think about the universe to how you go to the bathroom. It runs your mind's operating system and controls almost everything you do and feels.

Your brain makes billions of calculations per second, and neuroscientists indicate that, with over a quadrillion possible connections (synapses), the number of possible distinct states your

brain can assume is infinite! You might not feel this way because
so much happens unconsciously, but it is true.

And while your brain regulates a lot of your bodily functions, most
of your brain cells perform the work of computations –
calculations and predictions based on input and memory.

This means that it's likely that your brain and mind aren't being
used to their fullest potential, which is why you binge eat. There is
likely so much more you and I could do if we train our minds
deliberately to harness its power. All is well; let's go to the next
topic.

Your brain is selfish.

The brain's most crucial component of your mind, consumes a
disproportionate amount of your body's total energy requirements.
It uses up about 20% of the energy in your body but only makes up
5% of your weight. And this is where we start.

It's not crazy to think that putting more effort into thinking will
increase this consumption. No wonder we get tired quickly when
doing hard mental tasks if we don't train. We ask many of our
bodies and use many of their resources.

It's hard to do this. Because of this, our brains and the minds they
control have come up with some shady shortcuts and tricky rules
of thumb. Now we'll talk about the main point.

Your mind is slow.

Based on the first two points, your brain is powerful and uses
much energy. As a result, your mind is lazy.

It's a must. In its current form, it would take too much energy to work through every single detail of every piece of input you give it.

You would waste time on every little thing "do I use my left index finger or my right pinky for scratching my nose? Arrrgghhhh!! So many decisions!"

Given our environment's complexity, living and staying alive would be nearly impossible.

What happens, then? Your brain shortcuts things. It gives your mind heuristics and rules of thumb to guide how it works. In a nutshell, your mind tricks you.

Not tricks like a con man would play at least not with motives of harm to you. But there are still tricks.

At the moment, binge-watching is a way to show off. It's not as important to watch all the episodes of Squid Game or any other popular, must-see show, from Bridgerton to Money Heist in record time as it is to let everyone know that you did.

For the new generation of Internet users who don't like being spoiled, watching the newest episodes as quickly as possible is no longer just a lifestyle choice but a badge of honor.

But being passive and lying in front of a screen for long periods isn't bad for our bodies. Experts think that binge-watching can give us a drug-like high and leave us emotionally drained at the same time.

Before you settle in for a weekend movie marathon, it's important to understand the potential negative effects of binge viewing on your brain.

The true explanation behind why binge-watching television is so incredibly addicting

Show creators would like you to think that you watch an entire show, from the pilot episode to the end credits, in one sitting because they are so good at what they do. On the other hand, the true explanation is buried deeper in your mind. Dopamine is released in the brain whenever we participate in an experience that brings us pleasure. A clinical psychologist at Masina Hospital, Mumbai. "The mesolimbic dopamine pathway is a key part of the reward system and reinforces this behavior. Think of it as the brain telling us that this feels good and that we should do more.

When we watch more and more episodes, this chemical reaction in the brain can make us feel like we're on drugs because we want more and more dopamine.

Even though giving up social interactions to spend hours hunched over a screen might seem like a victimless crime, Sardesai thinks it's a cause for concern because most addictive behaviors, like gambling and drug use, come from the same neurobiological process.

Even though watching the latest must-see show will make you look cool to your friends, experts warn that it can be bad for your mind. Research has shown that watching a lot of TVs can make it hard for the brain to turn itself off, which can mess up your sleep cycle. Long hours of passively consuming content in front of the screen can also lead to cognitive decline, making you tired and slowing down your ability to process information.

Matthew Schneier, a writer for the New York Times, coined the term "post-binge malaise" to describe how people feel after watching too much TV.

This is because the number of people who feel sad after finishing a show is on the rise. Experts say that when a TV show ends, we can feel like we've been abandoned, empty, and sad because there won't be any more episodes.

This is further underscored by the emotional exhaustion from engaging with a set of fictional characters while bingeing a show. "Our brain processes all experiences similarly whether it is real-life events, books, or imaginary incidents onscreen," Sardesai elucidates.

A psychological coach in London named Lucy Spicer agrees. "Besides getting emotionally involved in the characters' stories, high levels of drama and suspense can raise our cortisol and empathetic stress levels, leaving us emotionally spent by the time we get to the last episode," she says.

Bing and dopamine.

There are about 100 neurotransmitters in our brains, each doing something different.

Dopamine is a neurotransmitter. It sends messages to neurons, which then make pathways in our brains. Neural pathways are the roads in our brains that help us remember how to do things.

One of the main jobs of dopamine is to get the brain to move by making it look for pleasure and then giving us a drop of dopamine when we find it.

Two of our most pleasurable activities are eating and having sex. Dopamine ensures we keep repeating these activities because they're enjoyable, and we need to do it to maintain the human race.

Dopamine can also be made by just thinking about food, even if you are not hungry. For example, you walk past a bakery and smell freshly baked bread. You think about putting a big piece of butter on warm bread. Your mouth starts to water, and you might even feel your stomach growl. The dopamine tells you to want the bread, and you start to crave having the bread. You can ignore the craving or go to the bakery and buy the loaf. You might want to buy a freshly baked loaf from reading this sentence.

The heuristic Effect is the first mind trick.

You might have heard the advice not to make decisions based on feelings but instead on logic. That would be just awesome if you were a Vulcan or an abacus. But you are not. You're a person. And human minds have a very powerful tendency to judge situations, concepts, ideas, food, and even other people based on how they make us feel. That is, what Effect they have on us. Or, as psychologists say, what they do. The affect heuristic is the name for this tendency.

Heuristics are ways to think quickly. They help us decide quickly about a situation, especially when we don't have enough information to do a thorough analysis. Daniel Kahneman, the Nobel Prize in Economic Science recipient, discusses this topic in his book Thinking Fast and Slow. He stated that

Heuristic is a technical term for a simple method that helps find good, but not always perfect, answers to hard questions – Daniel Kahneman.

Since my heart beat faster, this must be love.

How Emotions are Made, a book by Dr. Lisa Barrett is both wise and sharp. In it, she talks about an experience of affect. She had been on a date when she was still single. Before, she didn't find him particularly attractive. During the date, however, she felt her heartbeat speed up, she blushed a few times, and she even had butterflies in her stomach. She thinks to herself, "I must be interested in him."

After the date, she went home, threw up violently, and got sick with the flu. She stayed in bed for a few days.

This trick made her mistakenly think that her excitement (affect) was caused by her date. On the other hand, it was just a flu virus that made her immune system react.

Dr. Barrett doesn't say this in her story, but if the date didn't go anywhere, she might have told him, "It's not you. It's the flu."

Confirmation bias is the second mind trick.
Imagine that you were starting a new job, and a friend who has worked at the company for a long time pulled you aside and told you to watch out for Barbara. She tells you that she is a real b@#$h. She is also the boss, so you should avoid her to be safe.

Let's say you met Barb in the elevator on your first day. You say hello, and Barb doesn't say anything until you get off the elevator at your floor, and she goes to the so-called "ivory tower floor." What do you think about Barb? Was she not interested? Cold? Snobbish?

Now imagine the opposite: your veteran friend told you that Barb was a real leader, helpful and easy to talk to, and a real class act.

What do you think about the ride in the elevator now? Was she
going to an important meeting and needed to pay attention?

What's different? That, my friend, is an example of confirmation
bias. And it is very hard to get rid of.

Strong, but not too much

Confirmation bias is the one trick of the mind that has secretly
caused much harm.

Confirmation bias is the tendency of our minds to see new
information through the lens of what we already think. It is a big
reason we are so bad at being completely uninterested and
objective. It's one of the most sneaky things the mind can do.

This trick might be a way for your brain to protect itself. Keeping a
coherent worldview is important for our sanity and brains to make
accurate predictions. This is a good thing and is helped by
confirmation bias. Only when it's not.

We find it hard to change our minds at these times because we
have built up a false pile of "evidence" to back up our points of
view. The problem is that these pieces of evidence have been
tainted by confirmation bias, which is also true of your "evidence"
about Barb's personality. And voila! You've been had. All by
yourself.

Jumping on the bandwagon

We need each other. Our cultures, rules, friends, and neighbors
greatly affect our thoughts. This makes us vulnerable to mind

tricks from taking lazy mental shortcuts. The bandwagon fallacy is an important example of this kind of trick.

It just means we think that if many people believe something, it must be true. And if it's true, we might as well go along with the crowd.

We often follow the crowd when we don't know enough or have enough experience to make a good choice. Then, we use the social data of other people's experiences as a quick and dirty way to get around the problem. Since that restaurant is always full, you can ensure the food is good. If there are so many good reviews of that product online, it must be good. Right? Whether right or not, our minds make us think it is.

Marketers often use the word "best-selling" to get us to believe in their products by making us think of the "bandwagon effect." Most popular books sell more copies because, well, they are popular. It makes sense. Just one problem: because many people believe something, that doesn't mean it's true or even makes sense, either in general or for you. And the bandwagon can help us make important decisions, but it can't be the most important thing we think about.

When we have other ways to get important information, sometimes the best thing we can do is wave as the busy bandwagon goes by.

The bandwagon fallacy is the result of a lazy mind taking a shortcut. It can help us make simple daily decisions but shouldn't be used for important ones.

BRAIN FROM THE STONE AGE IN A MODERN WORLD

Dopamine also plays a part in how we remember things. More dopamine is sent to the hippocampus when a person sees or hears something for the first time.

Your brain is set up to remember things differently from what you've done before.

This is because it's good to learn new things. The brain decides if the new experience is important enough to remember for survival in the future. Also, the oldest part of our brain thinks that sex and foods high in fat are important for survival.

Back when we were hunters and gatherers, having fat stores helped us get through the winter and kept us warm.

Our brains don't know that the world has changed and that we no longer need to store fat to stay warm because we have central heating and onesies.

In the same way, when we were hunter-gatherers, being sexually aroused by a new partner would have made us want to mate and add to the gene pool.

Our primitive brains don't know that we already have enough variety. In today's world, our brains are constantly bombarded with new and different images, which advertisers and those who give us new and different pornographic images on the Internet use to their advantage.

Cravings

Every time you give in to a craving, whether for porn, a sugary cupcake, or a glass of wine, you strengthen that particular reward system in your brain.

When you look at porn or eat a cupcake, the path in your brain that makes you feel good gets stronger, and reward pathways that you don't use as much start to disappear.

Unfortunately, the reward system doesn't give you as much pleasure the more you want. The "novelty" of one glass of wine a night needs to turn into a bottle a night, or the porn you're looking at needs to change, or a "simple" massage needs to turn into something more. People addicted to sex or porn say they get cravings and feel like they are going crazy because their thoughts and feelings drive them to act out.

The only way to stop wanting to do something is to do it, so the addict stays in the cycle of addiction.

Bing and Other Addictions

Even though there are many kinds of addiction, sex addiction and binge eating are two of the most common and dangerous. These addictions have some things in common and are linked in different ways. Because of this, it is important to treat both of them simultaneously.

How sex addiction and binge eating are alike

Compulsive Behavior: Both sex addiction and binge eating involve compulsive behavior driven by the need to meet a psychological or emotional need. People addicted to sex or binge eating do these things even though they are bad for them.

Escapism:

Both sex addiction and binge eating are ways to escape reality and hard feelings. People who are dealing with stress, anxiety, or other problems in life can use sex addiction and binge eating as ways to deal with their problems.

Negative Emotions:

Both sex addiction and binge eating are often accompanied by bad feelings like guilt, shame, and embarrassment. People with these addictions may feel too ashamed and guilty to get help, making it hard to do so.

Negative Physical Effects:

Both sex addiction and binge eating can lead to a wide range of physical and mental health problems, such as obesity, depression, anxiety, and heart disease.

Triggers are things, situations, or feelings that can cause a person to act compulsively. Both sex addiction and binge eating can be caused by a wide range of things, like stress, boredom, and emotional turmoil.

People who have problems with sex addiction and binge eating find it hard to stop their compulsive behaviors, even when they know how bad they are for them. These addictions are often caused by deeply rooted emotional and mental needs.

Knowing how you think can help you get better.

When you wake up, the fog in your mind starts to lift, and all of your memories from the night before come flooding back. You pick up your phone and immediately start deleting messages you sent in the middle of the night and apps you downloaded the night before. You feel hopeless and ask yourself, "What was I thinking?" and "How did I get back here again?"

Cognitive Distortions

Working with the sex and binge addiction therapist, the client looks closely at how they act out and comes to understand their own triggers and faulty thinking, which we call "cognitive distortions," are a kind of cognitive distortion.

A cognitive distortion is a method of thinking that drives us to do something we should not do, whether we realize it or not.

Most of us have parked on double yellow lines at some point in our lives, thinking things like, "I'll only be gone for two minutes" or "Everyone parks on double yellow lines in this situation." Both binge eating and porn addiction are the same.

10 common ways of thinking that make people act out that clients have pointed out.

Rationalization: "Acting out is fine because I haven't done it in a long time, so it can't be an addiction," or "You can't masturbate without pornography."

Justification: "I can't help it when I'm drunk" or "No one could stop acting out if it was put in front of them on a silver platter."

Minimization: "I'll only be online for 10 minutes" or "It's not as bad as..."

Exaggerating: "I've had a terrible day, and I'm so upset that I can't handle it, so I need to act out."

Blame: "If my partner was more interested in sex, I wouldn't have to do this," or "If my job was more satisfying, I wouldn't act out."

Entitlement: "I need to act out because I didn't have much sexual experience when I was younger" or "I work very hard to support my family and deserve the occasional treat."

Uniqueness: "I'm a very successful person, so people would expect me to enjoy sexual variety," or "I was born with a certain fetish, and this is the only way to satisfy it."

Use a mental filter like, "The last time I acted out was great, and I don't regret it," or "My partner is always being totally unreasonable, so I need to act out."

Normalization: Saying things like, "All men watch pornographic movies," "It's natural to want to sleep with a beautiful person," or "Everyone wants to be wanted."

I'll never get caught: no one will ever find out what I do, or I won't get an STI.

Fixing our mistakes in thinking

Once you know your cognitive distortions, you can figure out when you first had that thought before acting on it. When we know our thoughts, we can act on them, ignore them, or tell ourselves they are wrong.

We often think we have no control over our thoughts, but we can stop and change our thoughts. When a thought like, "I've had a really stressful day, I need to relax," pops into your head, you can either agree with it and self-soothe with sexual acting out, or you can argue with it and say, "Yes, I've had a stressful day, but going to a massage parlor right after work is NOT going to help me relax.

I'll feel guilty and ashamed when I leave the parlor, and my marriage could end." Instead, I'll go home, put on my running shoes, and try to run 5k this evening.

"There's no softer pillow than a clear conscience," says a French proverb. So, if you don't want to wake up again feeling regret and hopelessness, become aware of your cognitive distortions and try to change them.

GOAL ACHIEVEMENT

Like the body, the soul gets used to any habit that one wants to pick up.

Your bad habits can hurt how much you get done.

Many people can't accept that what they do repeatedly leads to the results they see now. So it makes sense that habits only help a small number of people.

Goal-Reaching: Binge eating can make it hard to reach personal goals, especially those that have to do with weight management, fitness, and self-esteem.

The cycle of binging and purging can make someone feel guilty and ashamed, which can hurt their confidence and drive.

This can make eating well and exercising regularly hard, leading to frustration and giving up on goals.

When we want to do something, we often work hard to make some habits because we've been told that habits are the key to success.

However, when we examine how the various parts of our brains function, we discover that bad habits hinder rather than help us achieve our goals.

When we do things we're used to, we use our primitive brain, which is not the best for getting things done.

As discussed in the last chapter, the primitive part of the human brain, also called the limbic system, has changed over millions of years. Our ancestors had three clear goals to remember if they wanted to stay alive. These were the goals:

- Get food
- Meet someone.
- Keep away from dangerous animals.

The only thing humans had going for them was their superior intelligence. We weren't as strong or fast as other animals, nor did we have sharp teeth. The early brain evolved in a way that helped us do these three things.

When we saw that there might be food, we got a lot of energy, which made us want to go after the food.

When the chance to have children came up, we felt a strong desire, and when we felt like we had worked too hard, we felt the need to rest.

So, our primitive brain always tells us to look for food and sexual pleasure. It also tells us to rest instead of getting us to work out.

On the other hand, the modern brain tells us to keep ourselves in check.

Modern Brain

The modern brain, the prefrontal cortex, came about after people spent a long time trying to live independently. People decided that the three survival goals would be easier to reach if they worked together, so tribes were formed.

As people started to work together and in groups, they had to learn how to work together and in sync. This meant they had to learn to control some of their actions. People came up with social rules, such as:

Don't put a lid on someone else's food.
Do not take someone else's mate.
Respect other people's homes and don't try to take them.

We need a new kind of intelligence to make sure we follow these rules and don't break them.

This intelligence would control our primitive brain's most basic wants. Self-control is another word for the new kind of intelligence.

So, it's up to the modern brain to override these old instincts and guide us toward more important goals.

We must always choose between what we want now and in the long run.

It is up to the modern brain to think about how our primitive wants will affect us in the long run and make decisions that will help us.

So How Do Habits Hinder Us?

Habits are made in the primitive brain, so you don't have to think about them. When we try to use habits to reach our long-term goals, we are, in Effect, telling our short-term brain to take over.

And the short-term goals of the primitive brain and the long-term goals of the modern brain are different. So the result won't help us reach our bigger goals.

Try to make new habits.

While it may seem daunting to focus your mind on just one thing, like meditating on the Word of God, it can be a powerful tool in achieving your goals. The key is not to try to force yourself to pay attention but to practice word meditation.

Word meditation involves focusing on a specific word or phrase, often from the Bible, and repeating it to yourself silently. This technique can help you calm your mind, reduce stress and anxiety, and strengthen your connection to God.

By meditating on the Word of God, You may retrain your brain to concentrate on happy ideas and sensations rather than on ones that are unhappy or upsetting.

It's important to note that trying to form new habits can be difficult for our modern brains. We have a learning method based on rewards caused by positive and negative reinforcement.

For example, we develop a habit when we see food, eat it, and decide it tastes good. We remember how good it felt when we eat the food and then do the same thing again, trigger, behaviour, and reward, the cycle can be challenging to break.

Instead of focusing on forming new habits, try incorporating word meditation into your daily routine.

Locate a spot that is devoid of noise and where you may sit in complete ease and choose a word or phrase to repeat to yourself. You may want to start with a short session and gradually increase the length of time as you become more comfortable.

As you practice word meditation, you may find that your mind wanders. This is typical and causes no concern. Merely recognize the notion and return your attention to your selected word or phrase.

In conclusion, word meditation can be an effective tool for changing bad habits and achieving your goals. By focusing on the Word of God, You can rewire your brain to think in a more optimistic way. So, find a quiet place, choose a word or phrase, and start practicing word meditation today.

Use your curiosity to stop bad habits.

In an experiment, researchers told people to be interested in their habits instead of making them do things like stop smoking. They told people to smoke and to be very interested in it.

One participant said, "Mindful smoking tastes like chemicals and smells like stinky cheese, YUCK!" She knew in her head that smoking was bad for her health. Her habit no longer held her attention.

We return to old habits when we don't use the prefrontal cortex. When we're tired, stressed out, or trying to make hard decisions, it's easy to return to our old habits. Curiosity helps us pay attention to what we are going through instead of trying to eliminate it (habit).

As it says in the article Using Curiosity to Break Bad Habits: "What does it feel like to be interested? It's nice. What happens when we want to know more? We start to realize that cravings are just feelings in the body, like tightness, tension, and restlessness, and that these feelings come and go.

These are small pieces of experiences that we can handle from moment to moment instead of being overwhelmed by a big, scary desire that makes us choke.

When we're curious, we stop being afraid of our habits and stop automatically reacting to them. We use our modern brains and can think more clearly and scientifically about our actions.

So, the next time you have a bad habit or focus on short-term goals, try to use your modern long-term brain and be curious about your actions. In the chapters that come after this one, we'll talk more about this further.

Individuals suffering from binge eating disorder are often embarrassed and ashamed of their eating habits, which can make them feel alone and want to avoid social situations. This can make people less likely to talk to others and give them fewer chances to make and maintain relationships.

Interpersonal conflict: Binge eating can cause fights with

friends and family, especially if they worry about how it's affecting the person's health and well-being. This may put a strain on relationships.

Trouble making romantic connections: Binge

eating disorder can also make it hard for people to make romantic connections. Shame and self-consciousness about one's body and eating habits can make someone feel bad about themselves and less confident, making it hard to start or keep a romantic relationship.

Reduced self-esteem: Binge eating can also cause a

person to feel bad about themselves, hurting their social life and relationships. People with low self-esteem may find it hard to make and keep close friendships and avoid going out in public.

How it affects mental health

Guilt and Shame: After a binge eating episode, a person may feel guilty and ashamed about their lack of control and the amount of food they consume. This can make you feel bad about yourself and lower your self-esteem.

Depression: Binge eating can either be a sign of depression or cause it. People who binge eat may feel sad and hopeless and lose interest in things they used to enjoy.

Anxiety: Binge eating can make you anxious and worried about your next binge, as well as about your weight gain and how you look. This can make a person feel anxious and eat too much, making it hard to break the cycle.

Social Isolation: People who binge eat may feel embarrassed or ashamed about their behaviour and may avoid social situations where they must eat in front of others. This can lead to social isolation, which can further worsen mental health.

Spirituality: Fasting is an important spiritual practice for many religions and can have various physical, mental, and spiritual benefits. Binge eating can make it difficult for someone to fast, as they may be consumed by their cravings and struggle to control their eating habits.

This can make it hard for them to do this spiritual practice, which could slow their spiritual growth. A positive outlook and connection with a higher power can make them feel hopeless and depressed.

Health: Binge eating has been related to a variety of health issues, including obesity, high blood pressure, heart disease, type 2 diabetes, and some forms of cancer.

Finances: Binge eating can be expensive because it usually involves buying high-calorie junk food and snacks. Also, the health problems that come with binge eating can cause medical bills to go up, which can be hard on a person's finances. Binge eating can also make it hard to keep a healthy balance between work and life, lowering productivity and income.

FIVE EASY WAYS TO BREAK BAD HABITS

Changes to habits are hard to make because they are already a part of you. When you do the same thing repeatedly, your neurons get used to it, and it becomes automatic.

Because of this, your brain doesn't have to work hard when you do your morning routine.

Bad habits pull you away from your goals like magnets. They stop you from growing.

Many individuals wish to put a stop to them. They are unable to change, no matter how hard they try. Their habits take them in directions they do not desire to go.

Because bad habits make people feel good, they are hard to break.

Dr. Russell Poldrack said breaking habits that make you feel good is harder. When the brain does something it likes, it makes a chemical called dopamine. He said:

"If you do something repeatedly, and dopamine is there when you do it, that strengthens the habit. Dopamine makes you want to do those things again when you're not doing them.

Before figuring out what works for you, you must try many different things. There is no one-size fits all formula that everyone can apply.

Here are some scientifically proven ways to break bad habits or at least make them less bad:

Identify Your Habit Loop

Whether devouring a pack of potato chips or procrastinating, you have one bad habit to bid goodbye to.

Charles Duhigg shared the "habit loop" concept in his best-selling book, Power of Habits. He said a habit has three parts: a routine, a reward, and a cue.

Once you know each part, you can devise ways to stop or change those habits.

First is to pinpoint the behavior you want to change or your Routine.

It's when you take out your phone and scroll through your social media feed instead of doing what you must do. It's when you need to finish something but take a long nap. It's grabbing a box of cookies when you should be eating salad.

This habit takes time away from more important things you could be doing. Getting rid of the habit that keeps you from getting better is easier if you can figure out what it is.

The next step is to start working out what benefits you will get from using the Routine. It's what makes you want to do it again. It is the pleasure you get from doing it.

Duhigg said you should try different ideas to discover what makes you want something. Discover your big why or reason. As you test, change things like where the habit happens when it happens, or what it is.

After each activity, write down three words that you think describe it.

What do you like about doing it?

Is it because of how salty the chips taste? The problem? How it feels?

Is it the talk on social media sites? The popular joke? The news from your friends?

Is it because you took a nap? How soft was the bed? How the room smells?

Putting the words on paper can help you remember the thoughts you had at the time. Once you know the reward, you can find something else to do instead.

The Cue is the thing that makes you do the habitual thing.

Habits can be set off by a certain time, place, thing, feeling, or person. Making a plan to stay away from what sets them off can help.

Many people want to stop eating unhealthy chips but cannot stop buying them.

"Out of sight, out of mind" can become a rule of thumb. It is easier to ignore when you don't see that craving. Limit how much you talk to it.

How you act may show how you feel. When bored, you might look at social media for a while. A few minutes will turn into hours. It distracts you and makes you less productive.

To find out the Cue, Duhigg suggests writing five things when the urge hits.

To get a clear picture, you must figure out the five categories: place, time, emotion, people, and what happened before. Follow what happens for at least three days until you find the pattern.

If your bad habit is spending a lot of time on your phone, study the signs.

Time: Do you do it at a certain time of day?
People: Are there people involved when you do it?
Emotion: Do you pick up your phone because you're angry or bored?
What did you do right before you picked up the phone? What action triggered you to pick it?
Is there always the same place in the house where you do it?

Once you've found your habit loop, think of other things you could do instead. You can test a habit by changing the thing that triggers it.

 If you don't know what needs to be fixed, you might try to fix many different things at once.

It's Not That "I Can't" But "I Don't."

In an experiment, researchers from the University of Houston told one group to say "I can't" and the other group to say "I don't." After the study, they were given a granola bar or a piece of chocolate. People who said "I don't" instead of "I can't" were more likely to choose the granola bar than the chocolate.

This experiment demonstrates the importance of word choice and how it can affect a person's motivation.

Change "I can't eat potato chips" to "I don't eat potato chips." It's like tricking yourself into thinking you don't do the behavior.

Most people are easily convinced when they say they can't do something.

Looks familiar?

"Try this out. "Just one beer,"

"I can't drink that,"

"Oh, come on, don't act like a child. One glass of wine won't hurt you."

"I can't. I can't. I can't… Okay, just one."
Rather than:

"I don't drink beer. My body does not respond well to it."

END OF CONVERSATION.

Your words have a lot of power. What you say tells your brain what you should do next.

Choose words that will help you out of a jam. Use the phrase "I don't" with extra care. Use it when you think it will help you.

Switch out the bad habit for a good one

It can be hard to stop something. Timothy Pychyl, a psychologist, said that to break a bad habit, you have to start a new one.

When a person develops a habit, the neurons in his or her brain start to move in a certain way. This makes the action easier to do. It's hard to break out of this pattern. To break the habit, you need to start a new one.

Your neurons will gradually create a new connection that will become a pattern when the behavior is fostered consistently.

Elliot Berkman, a neuroscientist, agrees that it's easier for the brain to learn something new than to stop doing something it's used to without a replacement.

When you decide to replace your bad habit, think about the activity for a while.

If you wanted to make some changes in 2018, think about them now. Expose yourself to the materials involved and educate yourself about the matter. By doing so, you are preparing your subconscious for the transition you are about to launch.

The longer you've had the habit, the more challenging to replace it.

Many people cannot stand the process. They give in easily to the needs of their bodies.

But people who are motivated enough to change are capable of succeeding.

Don't Take It Slow

"Take it slow" is a phrase many people hear when they want to break a habit. Cut back on sugar first, then fat, and so on, if you want to stop eating unhealthy foods.

But new neuroscience research suggests that taking things slow can make it harder to break a habit. People say it's best to work on several bad habits simultaneously if they are all related.

Do you often fall asleep while looking at your phone in the afternoon?

Or maybe you like to eat while you watch TV, which causes you to gain weight.

You can work on both of them simultaneously if you figure out why. The habit loop can help you with this.

Though they are two different activities, they are closely related. They both affect a certain area of your life and performance.

Taking on both simultaneously can make you stronger and more disciplined. You can always get better if you work hard and practice often. You can get to the level you want by being responsible.

Activate the Red Traffic Light in Your Brain

Nicole Calakos, a researcher at Duke University, taught mice to do things the same way repeatedly. These mice were conditioned to press the lever to get a treat.

They looked for patterns in the brains of trained mice and mice that had not been trained. They found two types of cells with about the same number of each. One type sends a "go" signal, and the other sends a "stop" signal.

The same lever experiment was used to test the two groups. The untrained mice are better at resisting because their "stop" signal comes first. While trained mice's brains turn on the "go" signal first because of the habits they've formed.

When behaviors are repeated, the go trigger becomes strong and activated when prompted. Reducing exposure to the activity can slowly reduce the capacity of the "go" signal in the brain. This is good for breaking bad habits.

When you tell yourself to stop, the "go" signal doesn't get as much boost. The habit becomes weak over time when the go signal does not activate often.

Will They Break You or You Break Them

Cultivate only the habits that you are willing should master you. — Elbert Hubbard.

Changing what you always do can be challenging.

It's hard for most people to do. People who don't give up easily can get through these things.

Your habits can help you out. They can speed up your work. You can be efficient in any activity you decide to do.

But habits can cripple your progress too.

Many people are crippled to reach their goals. They did nothing to stop the bad habits. They don't work out the part of their brain that helps them resist temptations.

The champions of the world are people who are willing to sacrifice comfort to win.

At first, it can be painful to break bad habits. But you become a winner when you train through the pain and suffering.

You can rebound and repair the injury that bad habits cause.

It's okay if it doesn't work out the first time. Allow your failures to inspire you to redouble your efforts, instill new habits, and seek challenges to better yourself.

When you confront your struggles, you become stronger and more capable of facing the next phase.

Before you know it, those bad habits are now part of history.

They're no longer in your way. They don't enslave you. They don't dictate your actions.

You should instead show the way.

MINDFUL WAYS OF EATING

Mindfulness is a practice from Zen Buddhism that has become popular as a way to calm down and change how you eat.

Mindful eating is being added to behavior change programs and suggested changes to how people eat. This article talks about mindful eating and gives ideas for how to teach its basics.

Mindfulness has become a part of our everyday language, but its true meaning is deeper than how we use it in our fast-paced, multitasking society. This word has become popular because it encourages people to be aware of whatever is the focus. It has become a way to get someone to take better care of themselves. In the same way, "mindful eating" helps us become more aware of what we are doing when we eat.

Jon Kabat-Zinn said that "mindfulness" means "paying attention in a certain way, on purpose, in the present moment, and without judgment" (. Kabat-Zinn created and ran the Mindfulness-Based Stress Reduction program at the University of Massachusetts Medical School from the beginning.

Based on his experiences with this program since 1979, he wrote the book Full Catastrophe Living in 1990 to help people live more mindfully.

Mindfulness has helped thousands of people live more purposefully and to learn the skills they need to deal with chronic pain, illness, depression, trouble sleeping, and anxiety.

It has also become the focus of a way of eating that meets the criteria needed to change how a person eats.

Humans have long understood that a diet is useless if it doesn't change how people act. Even though we spend a lot of time studying diets to find out which one works best, we always come up with the same answer: all of them work in the short term but not in the long term.

Mindful eating entails paying close attention to our meals on purpose, moment by moment, and without judgment.

It is an approach to food that focuses on people's sensory awareness of the food and their experience of the food. It doesn't depend much on calories, carbs, fat, or protein.

The goal of mindful eating is not to lose weight, yet people who follow this technique are likely to lose weight.

The goal is to help people relish the moment and the food by encouraging them to be fully present during the dining experience.

Diets usually have rules about what to eat, how much, and what not to eat. These rules are meant to measure certain results. These outcomes are most likely weight loss or, in the case of diabetes, improved blood glucose values and, ultimately, improved A1C.

All diets have the potential for success or failure based on weight outcomes. People may know that their results will depend on how many calories they eat and how many they burn.

They may understand that this has to do with their behavior, but it is rare for people to change their behavior without seeing results in their results. Their behavior change will be subject to daily stress and outside pressures and, therefore, difficult to sustain.

Mindfulness is a behavior that is more about the process than the results.

It is based on what a person is going through at the time. The person focuses on enjoying the food experience and isn't worried about how much they eat.

The person who eats decides what to eat and how much to eat. It's not a coincidence that when someone takes a mindful approach, they often choose to eat less, enjoy their food more, and choose foods that are good for their health.

Many people who do mindfulness meditation and an increasing number of health professionals are starting to think that mindful eating can help people with diabetes change how they eat.

Diabetes education programs are recommending mindfulness more and more to help people change how they eat.

Even though I do mindfulness meditation and believe in the benefits of mindful eating, it's important to remember the results of a 2015 study.

Olson and Emery looked at 19 studies that mindfully looked at diet. Even though 13 of the 19 studies showed significant weight loss, the researchers could not prove a link between mindful eating and weight loss.

They suggested that more research be done to find the exact link between mindful eating and weight loss.

This suggests that mindful eating is probably linked to weight loss, but more research is needed to determine how the two are linked.

As was already said, most weight-loss diets work in the short term, but many fail in the long term.

What makes a diet like this work or not work? Successful people have one trait: they pay attention to their nutrition and keep to it, no matter the plan.

It may seem obvious, but this is the difference between eating "mindlessly" and eating with awareness.

Our advice has always been to pay attention to what you are eating, like "Don't watch TV while you eat," "Serve the right amount," "Chew 32 times before swallowing," and "Sit down while you eat." The point of these suggestions has always been to pay attention, just like when you eat mindfully.

Mindful eating is different because it is not about rules or guidelines. Instead, it is about how each person feels when they eat.

No one has the same experience every time they eat the same food. People should have their own experiences and be in the moment.

Mindful Eating in Practice

Kabat-Zinn helped me eat a raisin, which was one of the most powerful meditations I've ever done. Here is what I remember about eating raisins. I invite you to do this while you read about it or to read about it first and then do it yourself without reading getting in the way. Try this, even if you don't like raisins.

Get a raisin and put it on the table. STOP! Don't put a handful of raisins in your mouth at once. (Yes, there is a rule, but there's a good reason for it, which you'll see soon.)

Imagine that you were just dropped on this planet and have no idea where you are. You have never been to Earth or done anything there. You have no opinions, fears, or expectations if you have never done something. All of this is new to you. Take several deep breaths and try to relax.

Look at the raisin and pick it up.

Feel its weight.
Check out its surface, including the different ridges and shiny and dull parts. Really look at this strange thing for the first time.
Smell this object and notice how you react.
Listen as you roll the raisin between your fingers to hear what sound it makes. Take note of how it sticks.

Notice what you are feeling about this object.
Place the raisin between your lips and hold it there for a moment. What do you notice happens inside you?
Let it roll back into your mouth, but don't chew it yet. Just roll it around. Does it have a flavor? Do you salivate? What are your plans?
OK, bite down, just once. What can you see?
Start to chew slowly and pay attention to what each bite brings.
Chew the raisin until it is completely liquefied before you swallow.
Close your eyes briefly after you swallow to think about what just happened.

The raisin experience is a great example of what mindful eating can be like since the goal was to pay attention to different parts of each moment.

Focusing on how the food looks, sounds, smells, feels, and tastes make you fully aware of it in the present moment. This process doesn't tell you what to experience; it just suggests that you pay attention to what you are already experiencing.

The exercise is a good example of mindfulness meditation because it includes many of the attitudes practiced in each meditation.

Here are some attitudes that go along with mindful eating and living:

Nonjudging: When you start this experience, you'll first notice how you feel about raisins. Do you like them or not? We have tried raisins, so we all have opinions about them. To start the process of eating by setting aside our experience of the food is our first challenge. One important part of being mindful is knowing how we judge things.

Patience: To eat mindfully, it's clear that you have to be patient. Being aware of each moment takes time. Instead of the usual way of eating raisins, which is to throw a handful in your mouth, chew them a few times, and then swallow, you are dramatically slowing down the process to get the most out of it. You are letting the experience unfold instead of rushing through it.

Beginner's mind: When you look at your experiences like a baby does (taking one taste, one look, one touch, one smell, and one listen), you can see them in a new light and be open to what they mean in the here and now.

Trust: We trust ourselves more when we fully know our experiences and accept them as true. This is our experience; no one else's experience has to be the same as ours. By noticing and appreciating what we feel and our responses to different foods, we become more accepting of ourselves and, therefore, more trusting.

No striving: This is very different from being "diet-minded," which means that all you want to do is lose weight. Since no specific results are being measured, you, as a diner, can be in the moment and enjoy the experience to the fullest. Nothing needs to be done to make something happen; whatever happens to someone

is what happens. There are no expectations about what will
happen.

Acceptance: At the heart of the mindfulness process is learning to
pay attention to what's going on and accept it. This might mean
accepting positive things like the amazing taste of just one raisin or
more challenging experiences, such as our judgments about our
distaste for raisins as we place one between our lips. It means
being OK with whatever comes up in the moment. This is the
difference between being fully present and being distracted. It is
what it is.
Letting go: Mindful eating involves letting go of past
expectations, such as resentment about being made to eat raisins as
a child when we really wanted a piece of chocolate. When we let
go of things we've grown attached to, we can try new things in the
here and now without judging them based on what we've done in
the past.

There is a link between these attitudes; they are similar enough to
work well together. They are important in mindfulness practice and
are the foundation of mindful eating.

The other primary aspects of developing mindfulness are
committing to regular practice and intentionality. To be mindful
regularly, you must plan and do mindful things as part of your
routine. Examples include:

Mindfulness meditation is a sitting meditation that focuses on the
present moment.

Daily walking with awareness

Several times a week, eat with your mind.
Body scan meditation is paying attention to how your body feels
while you are in a meditative state.

Taking note of your breathing at different times of the day can help you become more self-aware.

By paying full attention to each moment without judging it and staying calm, any of these practices can help you develop a more mindful way of living.

The way to start this practice is with an attitude of intention. In other words, what's important to you? What are your goals for your practice? What will it do for you and your life to be fully aware of the moment? If losing weight will help you live more fully, that's great. Don't let your goal of being more present and involved in your life get lost in your desire to lose weight.

When you eat mindfully, you pay full attention to each plate or bite of food. It starts when the first thought about food comes to mind and lasts until the last bite is eaten and the result of the episode is felt. Some of the following ideas can help teach people how to eat more mindfully:

Before you reach for something out of habit, stop and think about how you're feeling and what might make you feel better. Are you upset, angry, bored, or sad? Are you by yourself? Or, do you really have a stomach ache? Be aware of how you react and choose what to do instead.

If your desire isn't to eat, do something else that fits the desire better.

Only eat what you plan to eat. Put away your other things and focus on what you're eating.
Besides how you feel about a portion of food, think about what it took to get it to you.

Who helped the plant grow and make the product? Consider the sun and soil it took to grow the ingredients, and ask yourself where it came from. Consider all of the efforts that went into creating it.

Savor each bite the way you did the raisin in the earlier exercise. Check-in with your body after each bite to see how you feel. Has enough happened? Do you want more? Should you stop? Then move on to whatever you choose.

Mindful eating is a practice that requires a commitment to behavior change, just like any diet or eating plan. Paying attention is at the heart of any diet.

It's important to say again that losing weight is not the main reason to eat more mindfully. But people who eat mindfully regularly will likely lose and keep weight off.

Mindful eating helps people feel good about who they are by telling them they are OK in a way that doesn't judge them and is self-accepting.

Education and help with nutrition

How to eat well: Everyone knows what they should do, but only a few of us do it as often as we'd like. The purpose of this book is to provide practical advice on how to eat properly while also explaining scientifically why most of us don't.

I'm not claiming to have the ideal diet. Still, my research and writing on behavioral psychology and habit formation have helped me develop simple ways to build and strengthen healthy eating habits without much effort or thought.

The previous Chapter discussed how our brain encourages us to binge. In this Chapter, I'd want to discuss why we consume the foods we do and what we can do about it. This guide aims to share the science and strategy you need to get the desired results.

Most of us recognize the significance of a healthy diet. You gain energy, your health improves, and your productivity increases.

 A proper diet also helps to maintain a healthy weight, which lowers Type 2 diabetes; some malignancies, heart problems, high blood pressure, and other health issues are all at risk. (Genes also play an important part. I'm not a nut who doesn't think genes matter.

But why is it so difficult to accomplish this when there are so many reasons to eat healthily? To address that question, we need first to study why we want junk food.

THE COMPELLING FORCE IN JUNK FOOD

Steven Witherly is a culinary scientist who has spent the last 20 years researching what makes some foods more addicting than others. A lot of the science that comes next comes from his great report, Why People Like Junk Food.

According to Witherly, two things that make eating food that tastes good is fun.

The first experience is that of consuming a meal. This includes how it smells, feels, and tastes in your mouth (salty, sweet, umami, etc.). This last characteristic, known as "sensation," is extremely significant. Millions of dollars will be spent by food corporations to find the most pleasing degree of crunch in a potato chip.

 Culinary experts will experiment to find the ideal amount of fizz in a soda. These ingredients interact to produce the experience your brain connects with a certain meal or drink.

The second factor is how much protein, fat, and carbs the food has. Food makers, in the case of junk food, are seeking the exact balance of salt, sugar, and fat that thrills your brain and keeps you coming back for more.

Here's how they do it…

Food scientists make people want food

Scientists and food companies use many things to make food more addicting.

Strong contrast: Several feelings are combined in the same dish through dynamic contrast. Meals with dynamic contrast have a crisp edible crust that is followed by something soft or creamy that is rich in flavor-active components., This law applies to many of our favorite culinary structures, such as crème brulee's caramelized top, a slice of pizza, or an Oreo cookie. That is incredibly thrilling and novel for the brain to crunch through stuff like this.

Response with saliva: Food causes drooling, and the more you salivate, the more it moves about in your mouth and covers your taste buds. Emulsified foods such as butter, chocolate, salad dressing, ice cream, and mayonnaise, for example, cause you to drool, which helps cover your taste buds with wonderful stuff. This is one of the causes for the large number of individuals who like sauces glazed in their food. So, foods that make you drool make your brain do a happy little tap dance and taste better than ones that don't.

Food breaks down quickly and loses calories quickly: Foods that disappear quickly or "melt in your mouth" trick your brain into thinking you're not eating as much as you are. In other words, these foods tell your brain that you are not full, even though you are eating many calories.

Michael Moss's best-selling audiobook, Salt, Sugar, Fat, tells of a conversation with Witherly that perfectly explains vanishing caloric density.

He hit the Cheetos right away. "In terms of pure pleasure,"
Witherly said, "this is one of the most beautifully made foods on
the planet."
"

I gave him two grocery bags full of different kinds of chips to try.
He hit the Cheetos right away. "In terms of pure pleasure,"
Witherly said, "this is one of the most beautifully made foods on
the planet." He named a dozen things about Cheetos that make the
brain want to talk more. But the one he thought most about was
how strange it was that the puff could melt in your mouth.
Witherly said, "It's called vanishing caloric density." "If something
dissolves quickly, your brain thinks it doesn't have any calories...
You can keep eating it for as long as you want."

Response based on the senses: Your brain likes variety. When it
comes to food, if you eat the same thing repeatedly, you stop
enjoying it as much. In other words, that sensor will become less
sensitive as time goes on. This can happen in a very short time.

Junk meals, on the other hand, are engineered to prevent this
sensory-specific reaction. They have enough flavor to keep you
interested (your brain doesn't get weary of eating them) but not so
much that your sensory reaction is blunted. This is why you can eat
a whole bag of potato chips and yet be hungry for more. The
texture and feel of Doritos are novel and exciting to your brain
every time you eat them.

Calorie density: Junk meals are meant to trick your brain into
thinking it is getting nutrients while not actually filling you up.
Receptors in your mouth and stomach inform your brain about the
protein, fat, and carbohydrate composition of a specific item, as
well as how full that food is for your body. Junk food has just
enough calories to tell your brain, "Sure, this will give you some
energy," but not so many that you think, "That's enough; I'm full."

You desire the meal at first, but it takes a long time for it to make you feel full.

Memories of food from the past: This is where the way junk food affects your brain and body hurts you. Your brain remembers how good it tastes when you eat something good, like a bag of potato chips. When you see, smell, or read about that food again, your brain starts to bring up the memories and feelings you had when you ate it. When you think about your favorite foods, these memories can make your body do things like drooling and watering your mouth.

All of these mechanisms work together to make processed food appealing to our brains. When you consider the science behind these items, as well as how simple it is to buy inexpensive, fast food anywhere, it becomes quite difficult to eat properly.

Make Healthy Eating Easier

Most individuals believe that altering their habits or behaviors requires willpower or motivation. Nevertheless, as I learn more, I feel that your environment is the most important driver of behavior change.

Your surroundings have a lot of influence over how you act. This is especially true in the case of food. What we consume on a daily basis is frequently determined by what is available to us.
Let me show you what I mean with an interesting experiment...

Healthy eating environment is important

Anne Thorndike works as a primary care doctor at Massachusetts General Hospital in Boston. Thorndike and her colleagues did a study over six months, and the results were published in the American Journal of Public Health.

This study was done in secret in the hospital cafeteria. It helped thousands of people change their eating habits without affecting their willpower or motivation. "Choice architecture" is a term that Thorndike and her team used. Choice architecture is merely a fancy way of saying that altering the way food and drinks are displayed has a major effect.

The researchers began by changing how the drinks in the cafeteria were set up. At first, there were three main fridges, all with soda. The researchers ensured that each of these units had added water, and they put bottled water in baskets around the room.

What happened? Over the next 3 months, Soda sales fell by 11.4 percent. Meanwhile, bottled water sales surged by 25.8 percent. Food selections were subjected to similar changes and outcomes. No one spoke to the people who came to eat in the cafeteria. Researchers just changed the environment, and people did what was expected of them.

Choosing architecture is even more important when you're stressed, tired, or busy. If you're already tired, you probably won't make much effort to cook a healthy meal or get in a workout. You'll take whatever is easiest to get or do.

It implies that if you spend only a few minutes today organizing your room, workplace, kitchen, and other locations, the shift in choice architecture might help you make better judgments even when your willpower is weakened or Built for sloth.

How to Eat Well Without Realizing It

Brian Wansink, a Cornell University professor, has conducted an extensive study on how your surroundings influence your dietary choices. Many of the concepts presented below are taken from his best-selling book, Mindless Eating.

1. Don't use big plates: Bigger plates mean bigger portions. So you end up eating more. According to a study by Wansink and his team, you would eat 22% less food over the next year if you made a simple change and served your dinner on 10-inch instead of 12-inch plates.

Similarly, if you're thinking, "I'll just eat less," it's not easy. The reason is shown in the picture below. When you eat a small portion of a large plate, your mind feels unsatisfied. On the other hand, eating the same amount off a small plate will make you feel fuller.

2. Use plates with colors that stand out from the food: Because your brain has difficulty discerning the portion size from the plate, when the color of your plate coordinates with the color of your food, you automatically feed yourself more. As a result, dark green and dark blue are excellent plate colors since they stand out against light meals such as pasta and potatoes, causing you to serve fewer of them. However, they don't stand out much against leafy greens and vegetables, making you serve more of them.

3. Put healthful meals on display in a visible location: For instance, you might put a bowl of fruits or nuts by the front door or another location where you pass by before leaving the house. You're more inclined to grab the first thing you see when you're hungry and pressed for time.

4. Wrap foods that are bad for you in tin foil. Use plastic wrap to cover healthy foods. It turns out that the old saying "out of sight, out of mind" is mostly true. Eating isn't just a physical act; it's also an emotional one. The things your eyes show you often tell your mind what you want to eat. So, you are less likely to eat unhealthy

foods if you hide them by wrapping them up or putting them in less obvious places.

5. Put harmful items in smaller packages and containers and healthy ones in larger ones: Large boxes and containers frequently stand out more, take up more room in your pantry and kitchen, and cause additional problems. Because of this, you're more likely to see and eat them. Smaller things, on the other hand, can stay hidden in your kitchen for months. (Just look at what you already have lying around. Most likely, it's small cans and bottles.)

Bonus idea: If you buy a big box of something unhealthy, you can repackage it into smaller Ziploc bags or containers. This should make it less likely that you'll binge and eat a lot at once.

There are two easy ways to eat well.

Most good diets have the same idea: eat whole, unprocessed foods that grew or lived outside. Some are unique (no animal products, no grains, for example), but the majority adhere to the basic "real food" paradigm.

The trouble is, if you're anything like me, you'll consume anything nearby, whether or not it comes from Mother Nature. As a result, the most effective technique is to surround oneself with nutritious foods.

1. Try the "Outer Ring" strategy: I only walk around the "outer ring" of the grocery store when I go there. I don't walk down the aisles. Fruits, lean meat, vegetables, eggs, lean meats, fish, eggs, and nuts are often found in the outer ring. These are outside living or growing things. I consume those items.

Things that come in boxes or are already made are put in the aisles. Don't go down those aisles; you won't buy those foods. If you don't buy those foods, you won't be able to eat them. Try it the next time you go shopping, and try not to make any exceptions.

Sometimes you'll need to go down an aisle to get spices or a bottle of olive oil, but this doesn't happen often. The last three times I went to the grocery store, I easily stayed on the "outer ring," I bet you can do the same.
How to Eat What You Want and Not Feel Bad About It

2. Don't fail twice: I believe that life is meant to be lived with happiness. I don't want to judge myself because I ate pizza or feel bad because I drank a beer. But I also know that when I eat well, I feel much better.

To keep the two in balance, I try to follow a simple rule: whenever I eat something unhealthy, I try to eat something healthy right after it.

It's OK to miss a healthy meal once, but I never want to miss it twice. Even the best people make mistakes but get back on track faster than most. That is what I attempt to achieve with my diet. I don't mind having fun and trying to enjoy life, but I also follow this basic guideline to get back on track with a healthy diet as soon as feasible.

HOW TO SAY NO TO TEMPTATION

Learning to say no is one of the most useful talents you can acquire., especially if you want to live a healthy life. Research shows that small changes can make it easier to say "no," resist temptation, and stick to healthy eating habits.

120 students were divided into two groups in a research published in the Journal of Consumer Research.

The only difference between these two groups was whether they said "I can't" or "I don't."

One group was told to tell themselves, "I can't do X," whenever they were tempted to do something bad. When offered ice cream, for example, they would say, "I can't eat ice cream."

When the second group was tempted, they were told to say, "I don't do X." When offered ice cream, for example, they would say, "I don't eat ice cream."

After then, each student completed questions that had nothing to do with the topic. As they had completed answering their questions, the students went to turn in their answer papers, believing that the study was finished. In actuality, everything was only getting started.

Each student was given a free treat as they left the room and turned in their answer sheet. A granola health bar or chocolate candy bar were options for the student. The researcher would note the food the student picked on the answer form as the student walked away.

61% of the time, the students who told themselves, "I can't eat X," chose the chocolate candy bar. When they told themselves, "I don't eat X," only 36% of the time did they choose to eat the chocolate candy bars. This simple change in language made it much more likely that each person would choose a portion of healthier food.

Why does a small thing have such a big effect?

The One Phrase That Will Make You Eat Healthily

Your words help you feel in charge and in charge of your life. Also, the words you use create a loop in your brain that affects the way you act in the future.

For example, whenever you say "I can't" to yourself, you create a feedback loop reminding you of your limits. This phrase means you're making yourself do something you don't want to do.

When you tell yourself, "I don't," on the other hand, you create a feedback loop that reminds you that you are in charge of the situation and have power over it. It's a saying that can help you change your ways to start doing good.

At Columbia University, Heidi Grant Halvorson oversees the Motivation Science Center. She explains the difference between "I don't" and "I can't" in the following way...

"I don't" feels like a choice, giving you power. It shows how determined and strong-willed you are. You can't choose "I can't." It's a limit, and you have to live with it. So saying "I can't" hurts your sense of power and control over your life.

"I don't" seems like a decision that gives you control. You cannot choose "I cannot." It's a limit, and you must accept it.

To put it another way, stating "I don't" is a psychologically powerful way of expressing "no," but saying "I can't" is a mentally depleting way of saying "no."

The most significant aspect of this is that changing your language causes you to change your way of thinking. You may now use your new, more powerful thinking style in all future scenarios. This is why a tiny alteration may have a significant impact in the long run.

Workouts and other physical activities
Medication and help from doctors
Therapy and help groups

HABITS IS BASED ON WHO YOU ARE

It's hard to change. You probably already know that.

We all want to get stronger and healthier, be more creative and skilled, and be better friends and family.

But even if we get a lot of motivation and start doing things better, it's hard to keep doing things differently. It's more likely that you'll still be doing the same thing next year than you'll have easily picked up a new habit.

Focusing on making a new identity is the key to building habits that last. Your current actions are just a reflection of who you are now. What you do right now shows what kind of person you think you are (consciously or subconsciously).

You need to start thinking differently about yourself if you want to permanently alter the way you behave. You need to make habits that are tied to who you are.

Think about how we usually make goals. We might say, "I want to lose weight" or "I want to get stronger" as a starting point. If you're lucky, someone might tell you, "That's great, but you should be more specific."

As a result, you declare, "I want to squat 300 pounds" or "I want to shed 20 pounds."

These objectives are results-driven rather than person-centered.

To understand what I mean, think about the fact that change can happen on three different levels. Think of them as the layers of an onion.

Change what occurs is the first step. This level is about altering your outcomes, such as if you want to have a book published, reduce weight, or win a competition. This degree of change is included in the majority of your goals.

The second part is changing the way you do things. This level is about changing your habits and systems. For example, you might start a new routine at the gym, clean up your desk to make it easier to work, or start meditating. This level is where most of the habits you form start.

The third and most important layer is changing who you are. This level is about changing your beliefs, including how you see the world, see yourself, and judge yourself and others. This level is where most of your beliefs, assumptions, and biases come from.

Results are what you end up with. What you do is what a process is about. What you believe is a big part of who you are. The issue is not that one level is "better" or "worse" than another when it comes to creating habits that stick and a system of 1% gains. There are advantages to change at every level. The problem is the way things are going.

People who want to change their habits start by thinking about what they want to accomplish. This brings us to habits based on what works. The other option is to build habits tied to your identity. With this method, we first think about who we want to be.

The Key to Long-Term Success
It's not nearly as difficult to modify your beliefs as you may suppose. It has two steps.

1. Figure out what kind of person you want to be.

2. Show yourself with small victories.

Decide first who you want to be. This is true for each person, each team, each community, and each country. What values would you uphold? What values and beliefs do you uphold? What do you hope to accomplish?

Although many individuals are unsure of how to start answering these major questions, they are certainly on the sort of outcomes they seek: six-pack abs, less anxiety, or a raise in pay. Start there and go backward from the intended outcomes to the type of individual who could achieve those outcomes; that is perfectly acceptable. What sort of individual could assist you in achieving your goals?

Here are five real-life examples of how this can work.

Want to get thinner?

Be the kind of person who moves around more every day.

Buy a pedometer to get a small win. When you get home from work, take 50 steps. Walk 100 steps tomorrow. The following day, 150 steps. If you do this 5 days a week and add 50 steps daily, you'll be walking over 10,000 steps daily by the end of the year.

Want to get better at writing?

Become the kind of person who writes a thousand words every day.

Small win: this week, write one paragraph every day.

Do you want to get strong?

Become the kind of person who never skips a workout.

Do push-ups every Monday, Wednesday, and Friday for a small win.

Want to make more friends?

Become the kind of person who stays in touch all the time.

Call one friend every Saturday for a small win. If you see the same people every three months, you'll keep in touch with 12 old friends all year.

Want your work to be taken seriously?

Be the kind of person who is always on time.

Small win: Give yourself 15 minutes between meetings to go from one to the next and always be on time.

What do you identify as?

It's far more crucial to show yourself who you are when trying to improve than to get excellent outcomes. This is especially true at first.

You can watch a YouTube video, listen to your favorite song, or do P90X to motivate and inspire. But don't be surprised if after a week you're tired of it. Motivation isn't something you can count on. You have to change into the person you want to be, and the first step is to show yourself who you are now.

This year, most people like me will want to get better. But many of us set goals based on how well we do and how we look in the hopes that they will push us to do things differently.

Stop being concerned with the outcome if you want to change, and start thinking about who you are. Make yourself the kind of person who can do what you want to do. Set up habits that reflect who you are now. Results can happen later.

Planning ahead and making goals that can be reached

Have a point. Set attainable goals. Get ready to make mistakes. And get support.

Find out why.
It's very important to know why you want to change a habit. You might want to stop binge eating so that you don't get sick in the future. Or maybe you want to lose weight and eat better, so you can do that. It may be obvious why you want to take action if you have high blood pressure: to reduce your blood pressure. You might be able to save costs on items you buy in excess or on medical expenses.

You must be willing to make a change. It's fine if you don't feel ready right now. You can still think about things and make plans. When you are truly motivated to change, you are prepared for the next step.

Changing habits isn't easy, but you can do it. Taking the time to think about what will motivate or inspire you will help you reach your goals.

When you want to make a healthy change,

setting goals and planning is key.

Try to reach small goals. Over time, this will help you reach bigger goals. With smaller goals, you'll be more likely to reach them, which will help you keep going. For example, you may want to lose 10 kilograms as a big goal (20 pounds). You might want to lose 2.5 kg as a small goal (5 lbs).

Put your goals on paper. This will help you remember, and you'll have a better idea of what you want to do.

Write down your goals in a journal or

notepad.

Put your plan where you will see it often to help you remember what you are trying to do.

Be clear about what you want. Having clear goals helps you see how far you've come. For example, it's better to set a specific goal like "eat one more serving of vegetables every day" than just saying "eat more vegetables."
Try not to attempt too much at once. Doing this makes you less likely to feel too busy and give up.

When you reach a goal, reward yourself. After celebrating your new behavior and success, you can consider your next goal.

Get ready to for the challenges ahead.

Trying to change a habit, do well for a while, and then run into trouble is normal. A lot of people try and try again before they reach their goals.

What are some things that could get in your way? If you've tried to break a habit before, think about what worked and what didn't.

By thinking about these problems now, you can plan how to handle them if they arise.

There will be times when you make a mistake and don't reach your weekly goal. Don't get mad at yourself when that happens. Learn from what you go through. Ask yourself what stopped you from getting there. When making changes to your life, thinking positively helps you a lot.

Get support

Get a partner. It helps to know that someone else is trying to make the same changes you are, like getting more exercise or changing the way you eat.

Someone is counting on you to help them achieve their goals. They can also help you see how far you've come.

Bring in your friends and family. They can join you when you work out. Or they can encourage you by saying how they admire what you are doing. Your family can help you eat healthier if they want to. Don't be afraid to tell your family and friends how much their support means to you.

Join a class or a group to help you. Most of the time, people in these groups face your problems. They can help you stick to your plan even when you don't want to. They can make you feel better when you need a pick-me-up.

There are also many online support groups.
Give yourself a boost. Don't waste time feeling bad about yourself when you want to give up. Think about why you want to change and how far you've come. Give yourself a pep talk and a pat on the back.

Get help from a professional.

A dietitian can help you eat better while still letting you eat the foods you like. A trainer or physiotherapist can help you develop a fun and easy-to-stick-to-exercise plan. Your doctor, a counselor, or a social worker can help you overcome problems, lower your stress, or stop binge eating.

figuring out and changing bad ways of thinking
Taking care of yourself by doing things

Learning to manage stress and emotional eating

Getting out of bad habits

In a 60 Minutes and Vanity Fair poll, 41% of people said it would take a near-death experience to break a bad habit for good.

But things aren't that bad. It's hard to break old habits, but it's not impossible. You can stop doing that bad thing by taking seven steps.

STEP 1: FIRST, ACCEPT THE CHALLENGE

Habits have half their power because we don't notice them. When we realize that a bad habit is holding us back, we must admit it is. It doesn't have to be dangerous to life for it to be important. It just has to get in the way of what you want.

If that's the case, say this to yourself now with as much conviction as possible: "I have a problem with [fill in the blank]."

No matter what's stopping you, the good news is that you're not alone. It's happened to other people, too. And because they were able to get through it, you can have faith that you can too. All you need is determination and maybe some help from other people.

Step 2: Figure out what your habits are.

After we understand a habit at work, we must understand how it works. This will help us stop being controlled by it. There are three parts to a habit:

The trigger. This is usually something we can see. But it can also make use of our other senses.
The way they act. We usually think of the behavior as a habit, whether overeating, putting things off or something else. But it's just how we react to what sets us off.

The prize. This is the hit of dopamine that the behavior gives us, which is more important than the physical feeling it gives us.
The trick is that we start to feel the reward at the trigger point, even before we do anything.

When you see something that reminds you of a reward, your brain gives you a hit of dopamine. It's like a credit card that makes you happy. The fun comes first, then the bill.

And this is where we go wrong. Why? Susan M. Courtney, a neuroscientist at Johns Hopkins, says, "We don't have full control over what we pay attention to." "What we tend to look at, think about, and focus on is what we did in the past that paid off."

So think about what you want to stop doing. Can you figure out what made it happen? Sometimes it's clear, but sometimes you have to think about it.

Step 3: Instead, say what you want.
Now that you've admitted you have a problem and figured out why it's so hard, you can say what you want. Some examples:

I want to find ways to deal with my stress other than smoking.
I want to work out five days a week and eat healthy, tasty food.
I don't want to depend on coffee to get through the day. Instead, I want to get more sun and sleep better.

The polar bear problem is a trick that people who are good at visualizing use. The speaker will ask the crowd to close their eyes and think of a polar bear in the arctic tundra. Then he talks in detail about the polar bear. He talks about its big, strong arms, vanilla-colored fur, big, black nose, and so on.

Next, he'll tell the audience to stop visualizing the polar bear. But they have made such a strong mental picture of it that they can't. When they try not to think about the polar bear, they can't help but think about it. Their minds don't want to let go of it.

The speaker will then tell them to close their eyes again and picture an eagle flying above a lake, looking for food in a place with many trees. He will build up that picture for a while and then ask a question no one would expect.

Who took the polar bear? The audience was shocked to see the eagle take its place.

Bad habits are like the polar bear in a lot of ways. When we try to break them, we keep thinking about what we want, and it seems we can't get away. But we haven't found our eagle yet, so that's why.

STEP 4: CHANGE WHAT YOU DO
We shouldn't try to fight our own brains. Instead, we should give them something else to do. The goal is to change the behavior while keeping the trigger and the reward. Consider smoking:

The trigger. You might be worried or see someone else smoking. You start looking forward to the reward right away.
The way they act. You light a cigarette and take a drag, which you usually do when you want something.

The prize. Your mind and body calm down.
Now, keep the same cause and reward, but change the behavior. For example, drink flavored water like La Croix when you feel like smoking. Or, take a walk. Or something else!

The idea is to find something you can do to shift your attention to something better and different.

STEP 5: KEEP TRACK OF HOW YOU'RE DOING
It won't be easy to keep the swap going. But tracking progress not only keeps your intention front and center, but it can also deepen your resolve and maintain momentum.

I suggest that you use an app to keep track of your progress. There are many ways to change bad habits into good ones.

I'm using HabitBull right now. It works on both iOS and Android devices, and you can set reminders, keep track of your streaks, and look over your results.

STEP 6: SEEK OUTSIDE HELP

If you need to, get help from outside sources. There are simply not enough positive things to say about it. There are whole groups that help people get rid of bad habits that hinder their progress.

It could be anything from a business coach to a personal trainer to Weight Watchers to AA. Name your problem and someone who has already solved it and is ready to help. Find them and use the knowledge they have to offer.

STEP 7: STAY ON TRACK
The change won't happen all at once. The last step is to just keep going. Keep at it until you get the results you want every time. It takes around 70 days of diligent work to convert a poor habit into a good one, don't focus on the timing tho.

CONCLUSION

In conclusion, binge eating is a complicated problem caused by many things, such as how the brain works, foods that are hard to stop eating, and bad habits. But with the right tools and plans, it can be dealt with. Mindful eating, in which you pay attention to your food and notice when your body tells you it's hungry or full, can help you break the cycle of binge eating. Binge eating can be stopped by using smaller plates, avoiding "trigger" foods, and finding healthier ways to deal with stress and emotions. It's crucial to keep in mind that rehabilitation is a process and that advancement might not always be linear. But it is possible to stop binge eating and develop a healthier relationship with food with time, effort, and kindness toward yourself.

BONUS: 50 Days Action Plan

For overcoming Binge Eating Disorder:

Day 1-7: Awareness and Understanding

Read your book and familiarize yourself with the causes and science behind binge eating.
Write down any personal triggers and habits that contribute to your binge eating.
Start keeping a food diary to track what you eat, when, and how you feel before, during, and after eating.
Reflect on your relationship with food and identify any emotional or psychological factors contributing to binge eating.
Day 8-14: Mindful Eating

Practice mindful eating by slowing down and paying attention to your food while you eat.
Try to avoid distractions like TV or phone while eating.

Evaluate your hunger and fullness levels before and after each meal and snack.
Use positive self-talk to encourage healthier eating habits and to challenge negative thoughts about food.
Day 15-21: Replacing Old Habits

Begin replacing unhealthy binge foods with healthier alternatives.
Experiment with new recipes and flavors to find enjoyable and satisfying options.
Use small plates and portion control techniques to help regulate your food intake.
Seek support from friends and family members, or consider joining a support group to stay on track.
Day 22-28: Nutrition and Healthy Eating

Consult a registered dietitian or nutritionist to develop a healthy eating plan tailored to your needs and goals.
Include nutrient-dense foods such as fruits, vegetables, whole grains, lean protein, and healthy fats in your diet.

Plan ahead and prepare healthy meals and snacks when you're on the go.

To assist in balancing blood sugar levels and minimize overeating, try to eat regularly throughout the day.

Day 29-35: Overcoming Temptation

Identify your biggest food temptations and plan strategies to avoid or manage them.
Practice stress-management techniques like exercise, meditation, or deep breathing to help reduce the urge to binge.

Surround yourself with individuals who are encouraging and supportive of your healthy practices.

Find alternative activities to replace binge eating, such as walking, calling a friend, or engaging in a hobby.
Day 36-42: Setting Goals and Planning

Set realistic and achievable goals for your recovery from binge eating.
Make a plan to reach these goals and break them down into smaller, manageable steps.
Celebrate your successes and acknowledge your progress, no matter how small.
Stay accountable to yourself by regularly reflecting on your progress and making necessary adjustments to your plan.
Day 43-49: Building a Stronger Identity

Work on building a positive self-image and strengthening your sense of self-identity.
Participate in activities that provide you joy and contentment., such as hobbies, volunteering, or spending time with loved ones.
Practice self-care and treat yourself with kindness and compassion.
Surround yourself with positive affirmations and supportive messages to help boost your self-esteem.
Day 50 and beyond: Maintenance and Support

Continuously practice the habits and strategies you've learned throughout this action plan.
When required, seek help from a professional, a support group, or loved ones.
Stay mindful of your thoughts and feelings related to food, and continue to work on building a healthy relationship with food.
Celebrate your journey and your progress, and Understand that Setbacks are an unavoidable element of the procedure.

Remember

Summary:

This book is about binge eating, a problem many people have. It looks at the different things that can cause binge eating, such as biological and psychological factors and environmental and social factors. The author talks about the science and psychology behind binge eating and gives practical ways to deal with it, such as eating mindfully, making new habits to replace old ones, and making healthy eating habits. The book also discusses how binge eating is similar to other types of addiction, like sex addiction, and how cognitive disorders and addictive foods can lead to binge eating.

Takeaway:

Binge eating is a complicated problem with many causes, including psychological, biological, environmental, and social. Binge eating can be stopped by eating mindfully, replacing old habits with new ones, and developing healthy eating habits. Binge eating may be like other addictions, like sex addiction, and it may be linked to cognitive disorders and foods that are addicting. People can work to stop binge eating and have a healthier relationship with food by making goals and plans, using small plates, and saying no to temptations.

Tips for making progress and words of encouragement

Hello there,

I'm so happy you've come to stop binge eating. Remember that change takes time and work, but it's worth it.

Adding physical activity and movement to your daily life is an important part of your journey. Physical and mental health can benefit greatly from exercise. It not only helps you get in better shape and lowers your risk of getting chronic diseases but can also help you deal with stress, anxiety, and depression.

It's important to find something you like to do. It could be as easy as walking daily or trying out a new sport or dance class. It is important to make it a part of your routine and stick to it.

Including physical activity in your regular routine might also help you modify your eating habits. Regular exercise can make you feel better about yourself and give you more confidence, which can help you choose healthier foods and stop binge eating.

I want to remind you that getting better is a long process, not a quick one. And it's important to always take care of yourself and be kind to yourself.

I know it can be hard to stop binge eating and talking badly to yourself, but I want to tell you to keep going. Do not forget that you are not alone and that there is hope for a happier, healthier future.

These pointers are what have worked for me.

Self-compassion means trying to talk to yourself like you would a good friend. Instead of criticizing yourself, try to understand yourself and encourage yourself.

Self-care means doing things that make you happy and relax you to take care of your physical, emotional, and mental health. Some ways to do this are to exercise, meditate, and spend time with people you care about.

Keep a record: Putting your thoughts and feelings on paper can help you deal with and understand them. It can also help you keep track of your progress and see patterns in how you binge eat.

Having a strong group of people to help you is one of the most important keys to success. Having someone you can talk to for support and accountability, like friends, family, or a therapist can make a big difference. I think you should talk to people you trust and who will back you up in your efforts to stop binge eating. If you don't have many people to help you, you might want to talk to a therapist specializing in eating disorders. They can give you the advice and help you need to be successful.

I want you to understand that you are not alone. Binge eating is a common problem, and many people are going through the same things. You can stop binge eating and take control of your relationship with food by asking for help, being kind to yourself, and learning new ways to deal with stress.

Don't be afraid to try new things; keep doing what you're doing well. Remember that every step toward better health and wellness is in the right direction.

I believe in you, so keep moving forward!

Last Word

Dear Important Reader,

We hope that you learned a lot from our book about binge eating and that it helped you get rid of this problem. Our goal was to make a complete guide about the different causes, science, psychology, and real-world ways to stop binge eating.

If you learn about the role of the brain, your sense of self, and even food addiction as causes of binge eating, you can better understand your situation and take steps toward lasting change.

People have been able to stop binge eating by using the strategies we offer, such as mindful eating, nutrition, and healthy eating, and setting goals that can be reached.

If you thought our book was helpful and informative, it would mean a lot to us if you could give it 5 stars. Your positive feedback will help us keep giving people trying to stop binge eating good information and resources.

Thank you for reading our book and giving us your support. We wish you the best as you try to improve your relationship with food.

Best regards, Georges.

www.ingramcontent.com/pod-product-compliance
Lightning Source LLC
Chambersburg PA
CBHW061507250726
48657CB00005B/1748